Animal-Assisted Therapy

A Guide For Professional Counselors, School Counselors, Social Workers, And Educators

Lynda M. King

A Master's Research Project submitted in partial fulfillment
of the requirement for the degree
Master of Arts

Ottawa University

February, 2002

Bloomington, IN 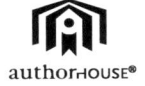 Milton Keynes, UK

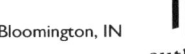
authorHOUSE®

AuthorHouse™
1663 Liberty Drive, Suite 200
Bloomington, IN 47403
www.authorhouse.com
Phone: 1-800-839-8640

AuthorHouse™ UK Ltd.
500 Avebury Boulevard
Central Milton Keynes, MK9 2BE
www.authorhouse.co.uk
Phone: 08001974150

First published by AuthorHouse 10/30/2007

ISBN: 978-1-4208-8662-7 (sc)

Library of Congress Control Number: 2006911200

Printed in the United States of America
Bloomington, Indiana

This book is printed on acid-free paper.

For Cody, my pet partner and co-therapy bunny

For my little spirit angels who have passed on

Acknowledgement

I would like to acknowledge the following people. I completed my graduate degree and my graduate thesis project at Ottawa University, in Phoenix, Arizona. Rodney Kirkham was my instructor at Ottawa University and guided me in the development of my thesis. A previous counseling director at Ottawa University, Ron Frost, reviewed and approved my thesis project. Tom Roche also reviewed my project. The illustrations were created by the author and Phillip Lansing. Phillip Lansing drew them. My portrait with Cody was taken by Life Touch Portrait Studios Inc. at JCPenneys. Michael Brown and Keri Smith took the photographs. I thank each of you for your own individual and unique effort that you contributed to my book.

"If we open our hearts to other creatures and allow ourselves to sympathize with their joys and struggles, we find they have the power to touch and transform us. There is an inwardness in other creatures that awakens what is innermost in ourselves." (Kowalski, 1991).

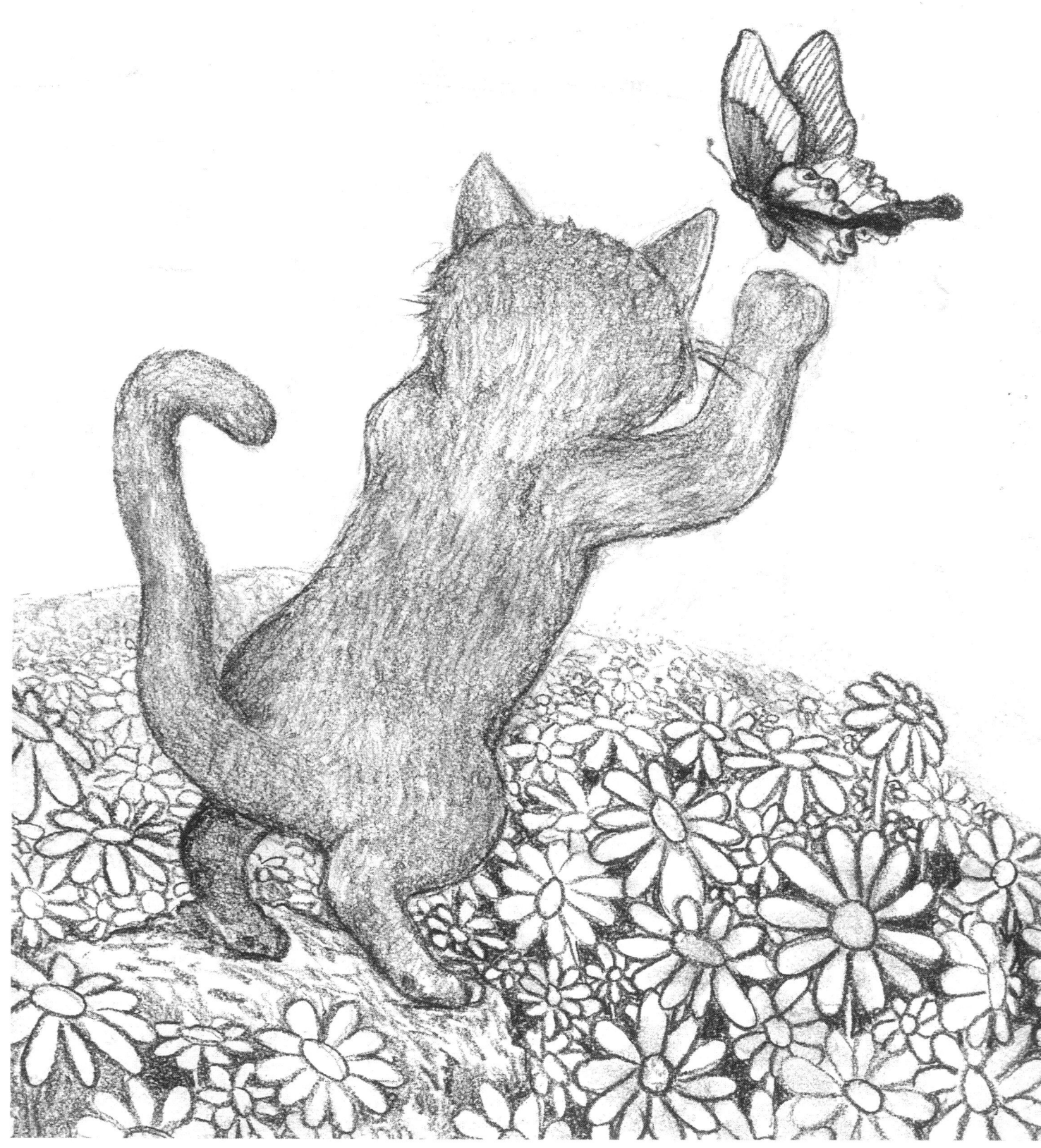

ABSTRACT

It is difficult for the client to enter a counseling office and begin sharing intimate details about his or her life to a therapist who he or she has never seen before. Animals provide an excellent means of establishing rapport, trust, and safety between the therapist and client. Animals of all kinds may be integrated into the treatment plan of the client and facilitate the counseling process. Animal-assisted therapy is considered an adjunct to the client's treatment.

Children relate especially well to animals, however, people of all ages may benefit in the presence of an animal. When animal-assisted therapy is integrated and implemented properly, the client, therapist, and animal all benefit from the experience.

This guide defines animal-assisted therapy and discusses the client populations who may benefit, as well as benefits to clients, the professional, and the animals. Facilities where animal-assisted therapy may be integrated are also identified. Some examples of animals that may be integrated as well as applications are given.

Tenets, ethical issues, and training and certification are included. Resources for the reader to expand his or her knowledge further in the area of animal-assisted therapy are given.

Table of Contents

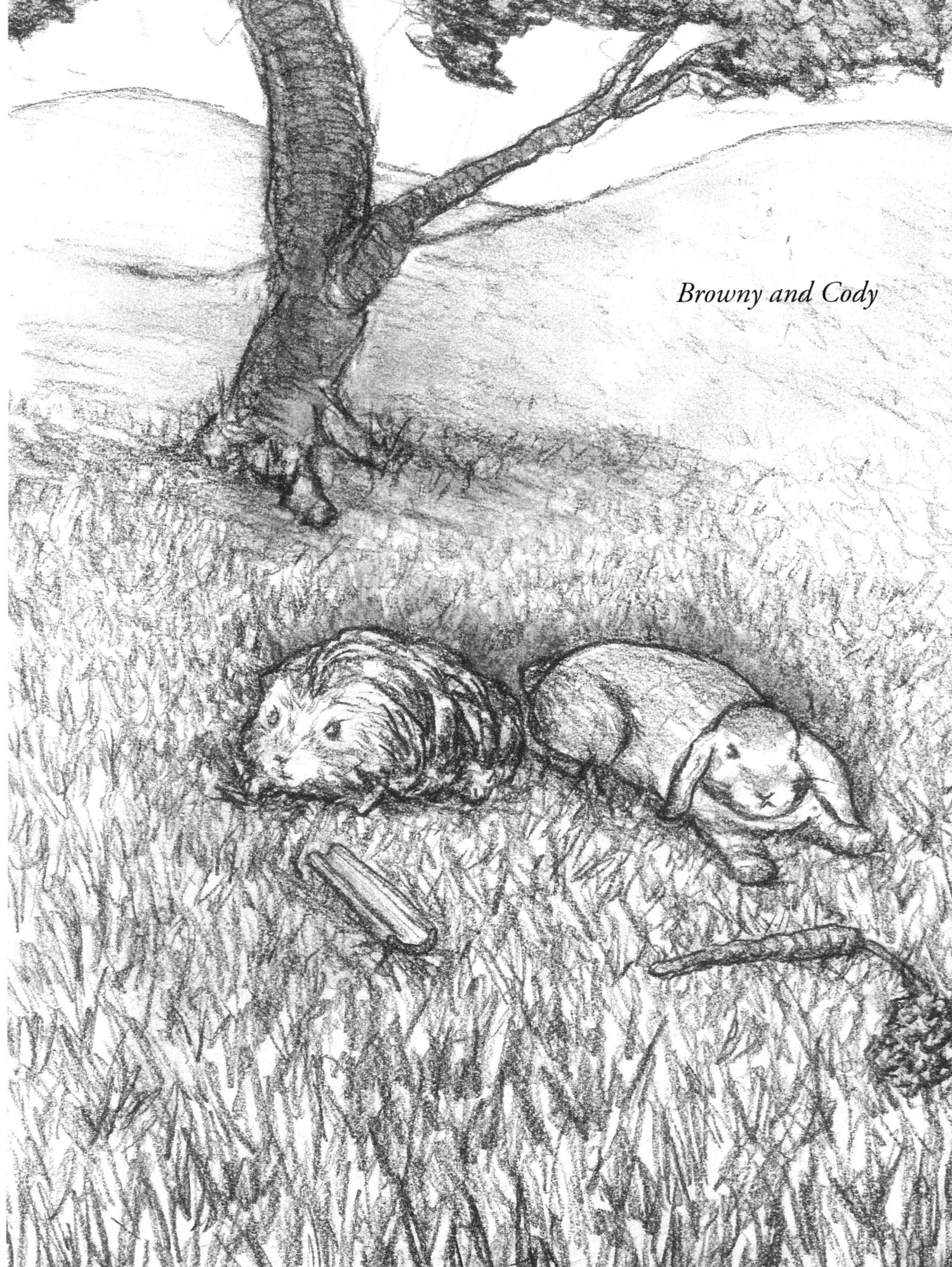

Browny and Cody

CHAPTER 1

THE PROBLEM

Introduction

Animal-assisted therapy has become a therapeutic technique that facilitates the counseling process. Animal-assisted therapy is goal-oriented, and uses an animal to help meet the treatment process of the client. There is literature, which is not consolidated, on the topic of animal-assisted therapy. The interested professional must spend additional time researching many areas in order to understand and learn about animal-assisted therapy. Animal-assisted therapy incorporates an animal into the client's treatment plan, which may positively affect the counseling process. All sorts of animals, whether domestic, farm, water, or marine, facilitate the counseling process in many different and beneficial ways.

The focus of this study was to develop a guidebook that will educate mental health professionals about the use of animal-assisted therapy. This guidebook will include the client populations that animals may be integrated with, benefits to the client and therapist, facilities where animals may be included, applications and uses of animal-assisted therapy, basic tenets and ethical issues, and training and certification.

This study is important because clients grow and learn through different therapeutic techniques. One of these techniques is the use of animals to facilitate the counseling process. It is hard for people to come into a counseling center and open up to a complete stranger, who is the counselor. Connor and Miller (2000) say that animal-assisted therapy can improve communication, foster trust, decrease stress and anxiety, and motivate patients. Animal-assisted therapy has been around for centuries, and caregivers realized early that patients benefited from the proximity, observation, touching, and tending of animals (Connor and Miller, 2000). Learning how to incorporate these animals into the counseling process is crucial.

There is a need for this cohesive guidebook because the literature that this researcher has found is sprawled out. This researcher has also found that the majority of the literature does not discuss how to specifically use animals to facilitate the counseling process with the client.

Development of the Problem

Over the last several decades, research had accumulated in the field of animal-assisted therapy. However, the data is not concise. The professional counselor who wishes to learn about the vast field of animal-assisted therapy will have to look at dozens of sources and areas to begin to comprehend each area.

The conceptual basis of this research study is that animals may facilitate the counseling process. The client may benefit in his or her therapy. Following World War II, Levinson, a psychologist, accidentally discovered the value of using a dog in therapy sessions with a disturbed child (Netting, Wilson, and New, 1987). In prior sessions, the child had remained nonverbal, thus, the child's response to Jingles, who was Levinson's dog, caused Levinson to recognize the possible benefit of using a dog as a communication link between therapist and child (Netting, Wilson, and New, 1987).

Since then, the late Boris M. Levinson, Ph.D. and psychiatrist, expanded his work in the field of animals and psychotherapy.

According to advocates of "pet therapy," animals can also make us feel better indirectly, by making strange settings or people seem less threatening (Vines, 1994). Animals can even promote social contact between strangers (Vines, 1994). Animals may provide comfort to a client who is anxious and uneasy about coming to see a counselor.

Animals are nonjudgmental, accepting and attentive, don't talk back, criticize, or give orders, allow people something to be responsible for, and offer a non-threatening outlet for physical contact (Burke, 1992).

Need for the Study

This study consolidated current and past literature about animal-assisted therapy. This cohesion will save the professional time in learning what animal-assisted therapy is, many of its uses, and how to go about the process. Clients learn, become motivated, trust, and open up through various counselors and techniques. The professional will gain applicable knowledge from this study.

Those who will benefit most include the clinical, school, and educational counselors, and social workers. The clinical counselor, school counselor, and counseling social worker can work directly with the animals in order to facilitate the client's therapeutic process. The educators can provide knowledge about the field of animal-assisted therapy to their students, who will practice in the field.

Purpose of the Study

The purpose of this study was to develop a literature based guidebook on the use of animal-assisted therapy for the clinical, school, and educational counselors who wish to incorporate animal-assisted therapy into their work with clients. Social workers who work within the realm of counseling and referral networking may benefit also.

Research Question

What is the content of a literature-based guide on the use of animal-assisted therapy?

Definition of Terms

<u>Animal-assisted therapy:</u> Animal-assisted therapy will be abbreviated as AAT. That is the most common form of abbreviation that the professional will see when reviewing current literature. AAT is a goal-directed intervention in which an animal that meets specific criteria is an integral part of the treatment process (Delta Society, 2001). Delta Society (2001) says that AAT is designed to promote improvement in human physical, social, emotional, and/or cognitive functioning and may be individual or group in nature. AAT is directed and/or delivered by a health/human service professional with specialized expertise, and within the scope of his/her own field (Delta Society, 2001).

<u>Delta Society:</u> Delta Society is the leading international resource for the human-animal bond. Delta Society has been the force to validate the important role of animals for people's health and well-being by promoting the results of research to the media and health and human services organizations (Delta Society, 2001). Delta Society's mission is to promote mutually beneficial relationships between animals and people to help people improve their health, independence, and quality of life (Delta Society, 2001).

<u>Water animals:</u> In the context of this research project, water animals will be defined as fresh water aquarium fish, saltwater aquarium fish, and other aquarium animals such as African

dwarf frogs.

Marine animals: In the context of this research project, marine animals will be defined as dolphins.

Domestic animals: In the context of this research project, domestic animals include horses, dogs, cats, rabbits, ferrets, guinea pigs, and smaller rodents such as hamsters, gerbils, rats, mice, reptiles, and birds.

Pocket pets: In the context of this research project, pocket pets refer specifically to the smaller animals that include hamsters, gerbils, rats, mice, and reptiles.

Farm animals: In the context of this research project, farm animals will include cattle, sheep, goats (including pygmy breed), chickens, ducks, pigs, roosters, peacocks, and other animals that would reside on a farm.

Wildlife rehabilitation: In the context of this research project, wildlife rehabilitation will include anything in the residential centers that the professionals and clients can assist with the care taking and rehabilitating of wildlife. Those included in this research project include eagles, hawks, and owls.

There are current trends in AAT. First, horses and goats have become known as domestic animals. Due to the literature content of this research project, goats will remain under the farm animal section. Second, marine animals and water animals have been included within the text and literature of AAT. Third, some residential centers have been incorporating wildlife and farm animals into AAT.

CHAPTER 2

LITERATURE REVIEW

GUIDE TO USING ANIMAL-ASSISTED THERAPY

Introduction

The literature in journals, books, and articles will be consolidated and integrated where it is applicable to the guidebook. Various topics will be presented in this chapter. They include the following:

1.   Client population.

2.   Benefits of AAT to clients.

3.   Benefits of AAT to clinicians.

4.   Facilities where AAT can be used.

5.   Applications and uses of AAT.

6.   Animal species used in AAT.

7.   Basic tenets.

8.   Ethical issues.

9.   Examples of animal integration.

10.   Becoming certified.

Client Population

Children, adolescents, adults, and the elderly may all benefit from AAT. Adults were included in the literature that this researcher obtained. The adults benefited from the animals just as much as the children did. Nursing homes seem to be the most prominent place where elderly people receive animal exposure, besides owning animals as pets in their own homes.

Current AAT literature has focused on children and adolescents, who both do well with the use of AAT which is integrated into the counseling process. Aaron Katcher, M.D., associate professor emeritus of psychiatry at the University of Pennsylvania, showed a correlation between animal contact and the improvement of a child's mental health (Golin & Walsh, 1994).

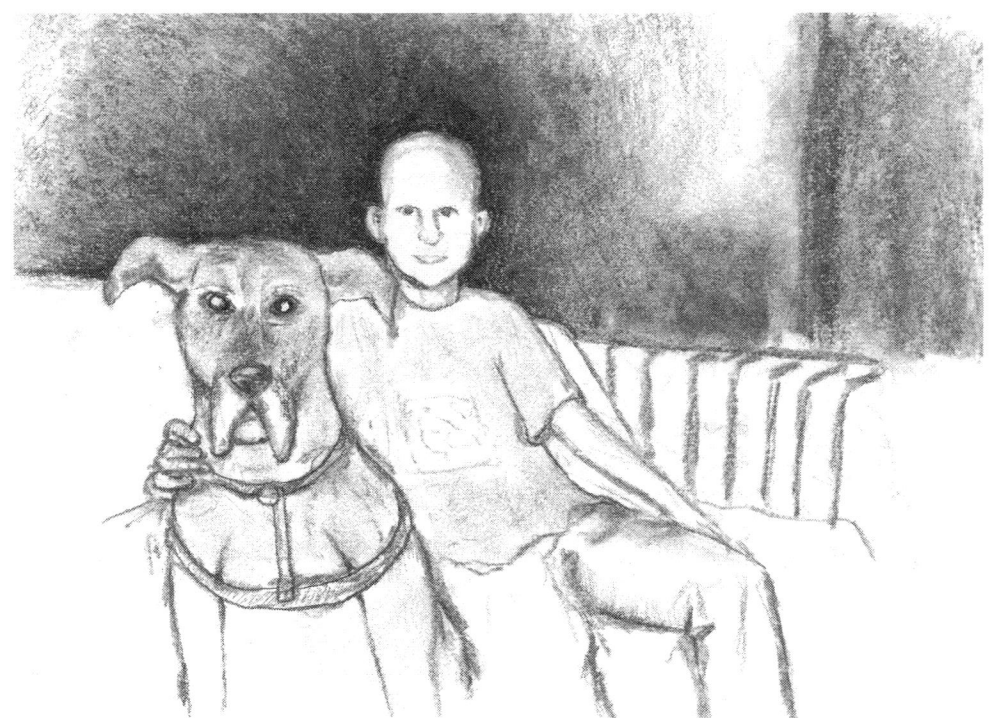

Benefits of AAT To Clients

Relaxation: AAT increases relaxation. Dzikowski (1998) says that the presence of an aquarium reconnects people with nature despite a sterile environment of plaster, walls, and fluorescent lights in an office environment. There's a wonderful calming effect (Dzikowski, 1998).

Comfort Level: The client's comfort level is increased. Kindsvater (1999) says that the idea of the pet therapy program is to boost the spirits of patients, as well as comfort family members in a hospice setting. Kindsvater (1999) writes that, "the dogs give comfort to patients and the family members, especially the kids," says Kantor (assistant director of development).

Trust: Trust is fostered and increased with the use of AAT. The children never need to fear that they will be rejected when they approach an animal, and as they are accepted by the animals on a daily basis, they begin to open up (Golin & Walsh, 1994). They relearn to trust people and not always expect the worst (Golin & Walsh, 1994).

Rapport and Communication: Rapport and communication will be fostered and increased with AAT. Dew (2000) says that Moses had initiated an action that allowed me to join with the client. Moses sat directly in front of the client, gazed into his eyes with his soft brown eyes and placed his paw on the client's lap (Dew, 2000). Moses is a two-year old golden retriever who assists his owner, a therapist, in providing co-therapy to her clients.

Learning and Acquiring New Skills: AAT affects the learning and addition of new skills. A research project is being conducted currently at the Colorado Boys Ranch, out of Denver. New Leash On Life is a ten week, animal-assisted therapy program in which boys learn to train dogs from local shelters (Dog World, 2000). The objective is to teach boys important life skills such as responsibility, patience and communication, while also saving the lives of abandoned or relinquished shelter dogs (Dog World, 2000). The project will be finished in 2002.

In another study, authored by Aaron Katcher, M.D., associate professor emeritus of psychiatry at the University of Pennsylvania, found that the exposure to the animals seemed not only to reduce symptoms of hyperactivity and what we call conduct disorder, but it also increased the children's learning capabilities (Golin & Walsh, 1994).

Home Environment: AAT helps to create a "home like" environment. Burke (1992) says that physically aggressive patients became noticeably more tolerant of people standing near them when an animal was present. As nursing researcher Robb puts it: "Animals normalize the environment and allow people to be more appropriate, more at ease" (Burke, 1992).

Physiological Aspects: AAT affects several physiological aspects in the client. Whitaker (1994) says that interaction with pets has been shown to lower the blood pressure and heart rate, subtle changes that have enormous health benefits. Bruck (1996) says that researchers have documented the therapeutic effects of pets, such as lowering of blood pressure and, most recently, a reduction in stress. When stress is alleviated, this in turn, will lower the physiological responses in the body.

Motivation: Motivation is enhanced because of the use of AAT. Connor and Miller (2000) say that AAT enhances motivation, the driving force that heals. Animal visitation and therapy in critical care helps motivate patients by reminding them that there's a life outside the hospital walls to which, in time, they'll return (Connor and Miller, 2000).

Green Chimneys Children's Services is a residential center that incorporates animals into the therapeutic process. The beginning goal was to raise animals and children together back in 1948, when the center began. "A very important thing that the children learn here is that if these birds, with all their problems, can survive, then so can they," says Dr. Ross. "If an eagle can live despite what's happened to it, then so can you" (Golin & Walsh, 1994). At the time, Samuel Ross, Ph.D., was executive director of the center.

Benefits of AAT To Clinicians

Stress and Burnout: There are several benefits that the professional will receive while incorporating AAT into his or her therapeutic practice. Stress and burnout affect many counselors. AAT was believed to benefit service providers by reducing stress and burnout (Carmack & Fila, cited in All & Loving, 1999, p. 3).

Co-therapy: An animal as co-therapist is less expensive as compared to working with a professional co-therapist. Dew (2000) says that she has always considered co-therapy an ideal way to counsel difficult couples or families, and yet it is not economically feasible for the clients. The use of AAT offers the client quality co-therapy.

Touch: Touch is very important. Many children do not have that. However, adults need touch also. Professionals are discouraged from touching their clients due to ethical and legal concerns. Animals allow the client to give and receive touch in a safe way.

Dew (2000) says that she has never seen anyone who instinctively knows better who needs touch and who needs space. She is referring to her golden retriever, Moses, who is her co-therapist. Dew (2000) suggests that Moses in his own instinctive way has no inhibitions or legal ramifications that keep him from touching.

Dr. Brook says that the domestic animals, including dogs, horses, goats, and the rest, provide something of particular importance: tactile stimuli (Golin and Walsh, 1994). Most of us were raised with opportunity to hug and to express love through physical closeness, but some kids here never had the loving physical contact so important to healthy development (Golin &

Walsh, 1994). Susan Brooks, Psy.D., is a staff psychologist at Green Chimneys center in New York.

Fairness: Fairness to all clients is crucial. Serpell, cited in Vines, 1994, p. 11, says that pets listen and seem to understand but do not question or evaluate may be one of their most endearing assets as companions, and it resembles the relationships some psychotherapists try to build. James Serpell, Ph.D., resides at the University of Pennsylvania. His field of expertise is animal welfare and animal behavior.

Dew (2000) also says that Moses greeted him (the teenager) and never noticed the teenager's external persona, but I did observe the client's physical appearance and wrestled within me not to make assumptions based on this client's presentation.

Facilities Where AAT Can Be Used

Out-patient and Private Practice: AAT may be used in an out-patient facility or a private practice setting. Brenda L. Dew, Ph.D., maintains a part-time private practice in marriage and family counseling, as well as associate and adjunct professor (Dew, 2000). She uses Moses as her co-therapist, who is very effective.

In-patient and Residential Centers: AAT may be used in an in-patient residential setting. At the Green Chimneys Children's Services in New York, mending birds' wings appears to rehabilitate the damaged psyches of the children as well (Burke, 1992). Director Sam Ross believes that the kid's identify with injured animals (Burke, 1992).

Hospitals: AAT may be used in a hospital setting. Bardill and Hutchinson (1997) say that a therapeutic milieu in a psychiatric hospital environment fosters the adolescent's functioning and sharing in community responsibilities, as might occur in a family. The less institutional and rigid the unit can appear, the better it is in preparing the patient to function optimally in the family and community (Bardill and Hutchinson, 1997). Spencer, cited in Janssen, 1998, pg. 40, says that on a children's cancer ward, Animal Assisted Therapy animals have been placed on beds with children who are tearful and cannot sleep.

Schools: Schools are a place where AAT may be used. Black (1996) says that in a rural school, two golden retrievers are the 'welcome mat' in the counselor's office. "Kids who haven't said a word to anyone for weeks will tell the dogs their innermost fears and secrets," says the school counselor (Black, 1996).

Trivedi and Perl (1995) say that at an elementary school, a small mixed-breed dog, Sarah Jane, is a regular part of the counseling program and contributes to a positive school climate. Sarah Jane serves as a companion to children who attend counseling sessions, and she has helped insecure or shy children feel less self-conscious and more comfortable in her presence (Trivedi and Perl, 1995). Trivedi and Perl (1995) also say that a reality of a dog unconditionally accepting children has produced an observable effect on the self-esteem of many children at our school, and Sarah Jane's presence in counseling sessions has helped many children to make marked therapeutic gains.

Hospices: AAT may be used in hospices. Kindsvater (1999) says that Nathan Adelson Hospice recently implemented a pet therapy program for use with its clients. "The dogs give comfort to patients and the family members, especially the kids," Kantor said (Kindsvater, 1999). Heather Kantor is the assistant director of development at Nathan Adelson Hospice in Nevada.

At Hospice of the Western Reserve in Cleveland, OH, Sally, the resident golden retriever, has an uncanny talent for knowing when she's needed and by whom, often seeking out patients without visitors, sitting her head in their laps or curling up on the floor next to their beds (Bruck, 1996).

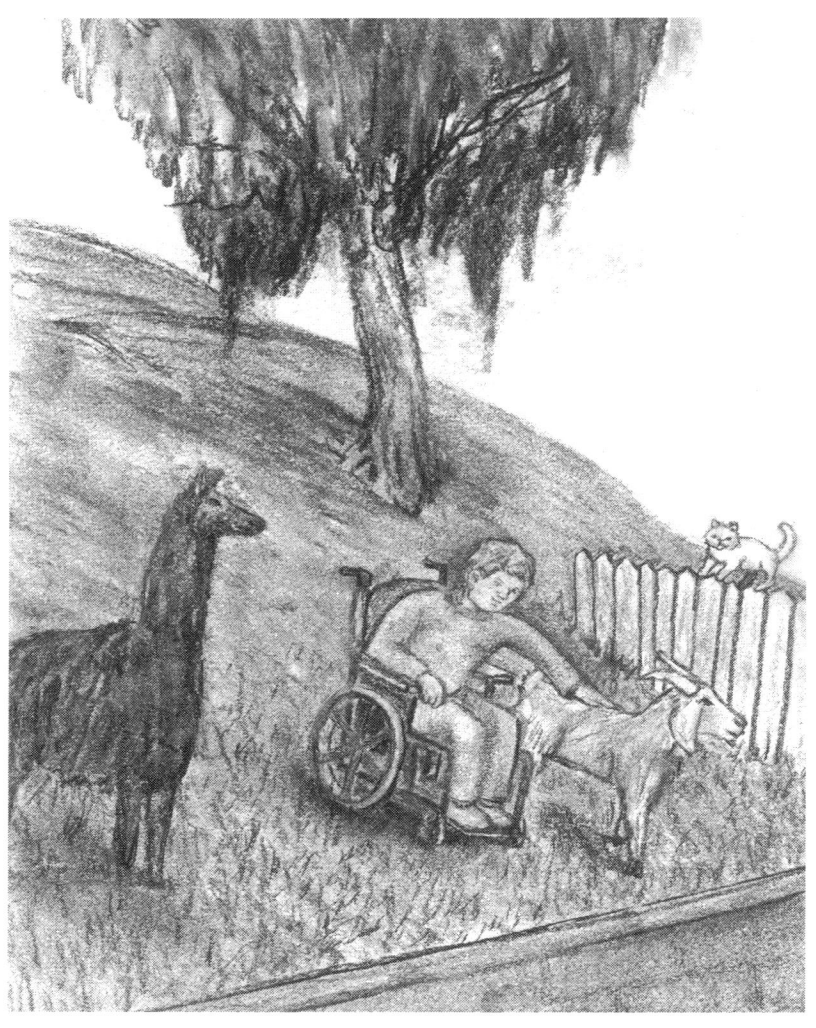

Retreats and Camps: Retreats and camps are places where AAT may be used. Some retreats and camps have specific AAT programs and others are less structured. Whispering Hope

Ranch, in Payson, AZ, offers a free flowing interaction with animals. The mission statement of Whispering Hope Ranch is to provide a place of beauty and serenity where animals interact with people to heal the body, mind, and spirit (Whispering Hope Ranch, brochure).

This program is for those whose lives have been altered by events, illness, or injury or who have lost their ability to feel love and joy (Whispering Hope Ranch, brochure). This program is for animals who have been hurt, lost their caregiver, or are physically different (Whispering Hope Ranch, brochure).

The animals seek out those people who need special attention. Nursing home residents, developmentally disabled adults, high-risk children, families, and individuals all come when they are in need of peace. Whispering Hope Ranch does not provide structured AAT, however people of all walks of life may benefit by visiting for the day. This would be a good place for a counselor to send a couple or family who is in need of spending time together. They offer camps for many special needs children. They also offer special programs for developmentally disabled children. These children may relate well to the animals who have physical deformities or have been abused previously. The counselor may refer these children to Whispering Hope Ranch.

Burke (1992) says that as far back as the 1790s at a Quaker retreat in York, England, patients were encouraged to spend time with farm animals roaming the grounds. The reasoning was that this pursuit would improve their mental state more than the archaic, sometimes brutal "therapies" commonly prescribed for the mentally ill at that time (Burke, 1992).

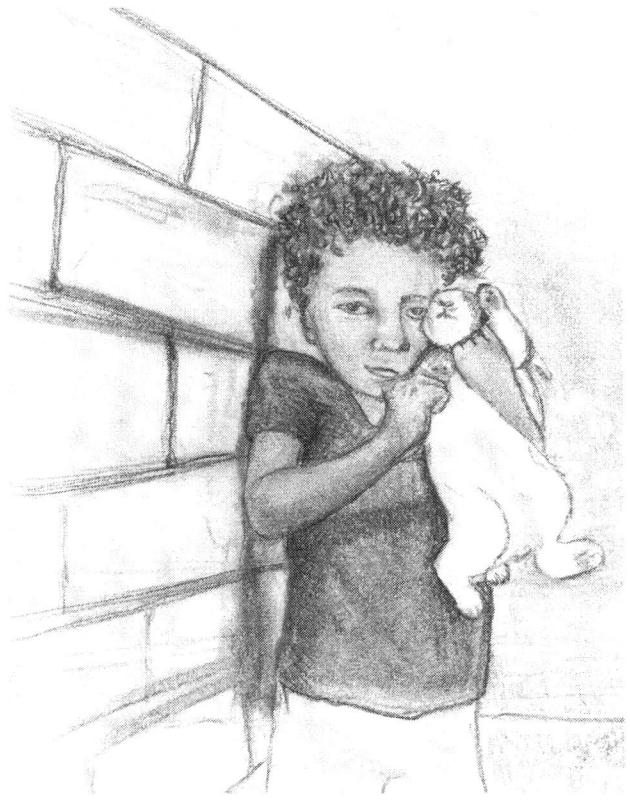

Crisis Intervention Sites: Crisis intervention sites are places where AAT may be used. A little boy around the age of five years old had been a victim in the Oklahoma City bombing and his baby sister was missing. The boy had quit speaking. Siegel (1995) says that Shellie, a dog, arrived on the scene, and began working wonders. The little boy scooped Shellie up in his arms and hugged her, before giving in to racking sobs (Siegel, 1995). A counselor watched and felt a sense of relief: "Now he'll be able to grieve" (Siegel, 1995).

Breeders John and Vicky McCuan brought eight of their rabbits to that same bombing incident. "A woman whose husband had been killed asked if she could hold one of my rabbits," recalls John McCuan (Siegel, 1995). "She walked around, hugging the animal," and said, 'I just needed something' (Siegel, 1995).

<u>Prisons and Shelters:</u> Prisons and shelters will be discussed together, because very little research has been done in these two areas as compared with the topics listed above. Shelters may include homeless and domestic violence.

Janssen (1998) says that dogs, that are part of a program called Unconditional Love, Inc. in California, provide animal assisted therapy to adults and children in their local area. These clients may be individuals with Alzheimer's Disease, inmates in correctional facilities, guests in homeless shelters, or youths at school or adolescent treatment facilities. These dogs provide therapy through specific goals and objectives (Janssen, 1998). In a double bonus, women inmates in Gig Harbor, Wash., are training special dogs to aid the handicapped (Toufexis, 1987).

<u>Animal Shelters:</u> Children and teenagers may be sent to volunteer in animal shelters. The therapist must determine whether the client may harm an animal or run away (awol) once they leave the residential treatment center, group home, or shelter. AAT may be used when the client returns to the place of residence.

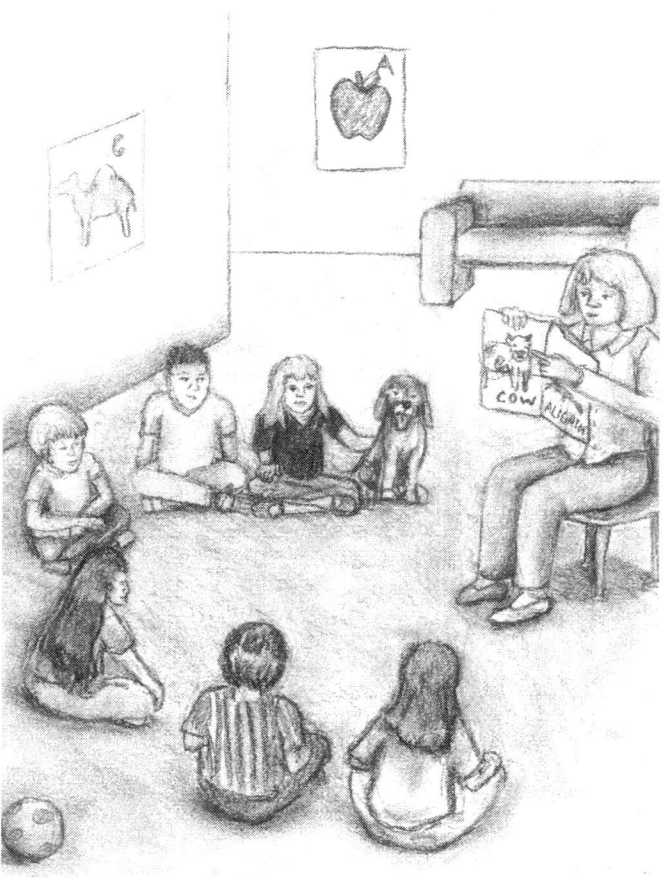

Lansdell says that the animals in this shelter and the students in my classroom showed me that when "throwaway" kids and "throwaway" animals give and receive love from each other, they form relationships and families that help them to survive (cited in Anderson and Anderson, 1999). Lansdell also says that the world may have forgotten about and not needed my kids, but the animals sure did (cited in Anderson and Anderson, 1999). These shining animals showed some very needy kids the way back home from heartbreak and abuse (Lansdell, cited in Anderson and Anderson, 1999, p. 89).

Applications and Uses of AAT

<u>Depression:</u> The depressed client can have animals added to his or her therapeutic process. For the depressed or despondent, the unique relationship with a pet may be a

necessary first step to recovery (Whitaker, 1994). Pet therapy has proved successful with medical patients suffering from depression (McCulloch, cited in Sable, 1995, pg. 2).

Loneliness: Loneliness can be reduced within the patient by the use of animal-assisted therapy (Connor and Miller, 2000). Easing the distress of loneliness and increasing interaction with animals and humans benefit the client emotionally and motivationally (Janssen, 1998). Pets may supply ongoing comfort and reduce feelings of loneliness during adversity or stressful transitions such as divorce or bereavement (Sable, 1995). Isolation can be reduced or eliminated by decreasing loneliness and increasing communication skills. Whitaker (1994) says that pets require that you extend yourself when you normally wouldn't.

Anxiety and Stress: Anxiety and stress can be decreased when patients observe, touch, and tend to animals (Connor and Miller, 2000). Dzikowski (1998) says that studies by the University of Pennsylvania and Purdue University found that watching aquarium displays can reduce stress and lower blood pressure. Jessen, who professionally installs aquariums, says "There's a wonderful calming effect" (Dzikowski, 1998).

Posttraumatic Stress Disorder: PTSD patients, who are often refractory to therapy, and indeed may tend to separate themselves from [human] society, may benefit from interacting with their animals (Altschuler, 1999). A patient with PTSD recently told me that his anxiety was much increased at times when he had to be separated from his pet (Altschuler, 1999).

Abuse and Neglect: Abuse and neglect have been some experiences of New York's inner city children who have been referred to Green Chimneys Children's Services (Golin and Walsh, 1994). They understand and relate to animals that have been injured or beaten up. They talk to the bird and tell him how sorry they are to hear his story, and then they go on and tell him theirs (Golin and Walsh, 1994).

Attachment Disorders: Attachment disorders can be improved upon through the use of animals. Pets can uniquely fill a combination of emotional needs, sometimes substituting for an absence of human attachment and at other times expanding the range of relationships and social contacts that add to the pleasures of life and give a feeling of comfort and companionship in times of difficulty (Sable, 1995). Attachment theory highlights the lifelong requirement for close affectionate bonds with others (Sable, 1995).

The substitute attachment of a pet provides closeness, touching, and a chance to feel worthwhile and needed (Sable, 1995). Sable (1995) also says that the animal may have special value for elderly people, who are apt to experience disruptions in relationships with familiar people, places, and things, as well as declining health, physical incapacity, and limited financial resources.

Self Esteem and Self Worth: Self esteem and self worth can be increased. The psychology behind the human companion animal bond is based primarily on three fundamental principles that all people need to love and be loved, need to feel worthwhile, and pets fulfill these needs (Janssen, 1998).

Grief: Grief can be alleviated or reduced through the use of animals. Sable (1995) says that a complaint of bereaved spouses is that social support tends to be mobilized at the time of loss but then quickly ends. Sable (1995) also says that one very unique aspect of pets is their constant proximity. As was stated previously in the crisis intervention site, the woman whose husband had been killed held the rabbit because she needed something during her time of grief. Touch can be significant during a time of grief and loss.

Interpersonal Relationships: Interpersonal relationships can be fostered through the use of animals. If the children can build a healthy relationship with a horse, dog, or bird, then that's a starting point for them to build a healthy relationship with their peers and then with the staff (Golin and Walsh, 1994). Dr. Susan Brooks says that they use animal-assisted therapy as the starting point to get the children to open up (Golin and Walsh, 1994).

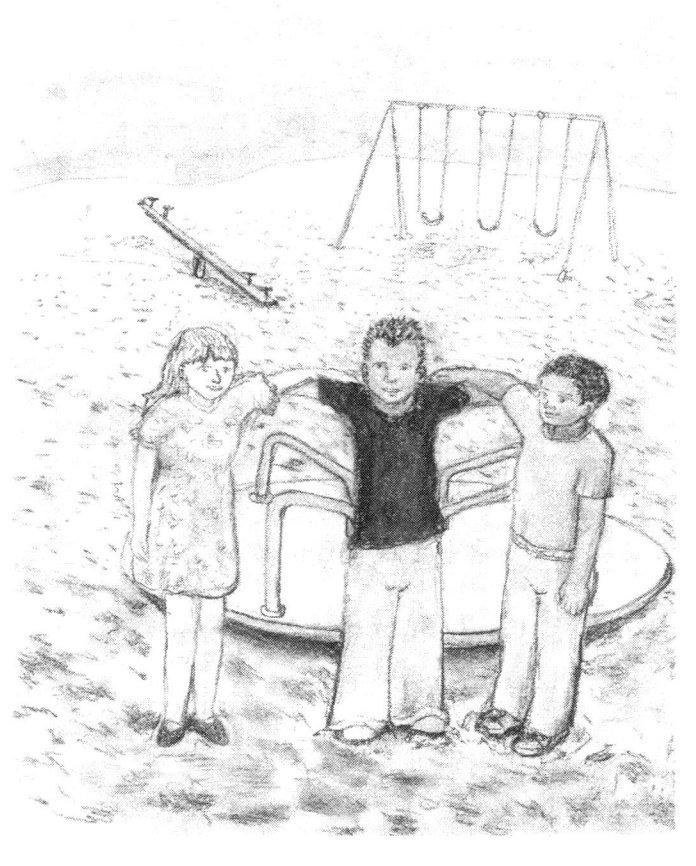

Appropriate Touching: In the book, Animal-Assisted Therapy: Therapeutic Interventions, the mental health worker can learn how to discuss and teach appropriate touching to children. First, the therapist can discuss how the animals feel when touched in different manners (Gammonley, Howie, Kirwin, Zapf, Frye, Freeman, & Stuart-Russell, 1997). Second, the therapist can discuss the appropriate areas of the animal's body to touch (Gammonley, et al, 1997). Third, the therapist can discuss the difference between a "good" touch and a "bad" touch (Gammonley, et al, 1997).

Conduct Disorder: Conduct disorder occurs among some children and adolescents who have been abused and neglected, to name a few. Many of these kids have simply retreated from the world (Golin and Walsh, 1994). The years of hardship have fostered such a long list of learning disabilities, emotional disorders, and behavioral problems that they can't engage in effective relationships with other people and can't function normally in a typical classroom or social setting (Golin and Walsh, 1994). "Exposure to the animals seemed not only to reduce symptoms of hyperactivity and what we call conduct disorder, but it also increased the children's learning capabilities," says Aaron Katcher, M.D. (Golin and Walsh, 1994).

Animal Species used in AAT

Dogs: Dogs are the most popular animals that may be used to facilitate the counseling process. Brenda Dew, Ph.D., practices co-therapy with Moses, her golden retriever as was stated earlier in this thesis. Their basic theoretical model is nonverbal collaborative language (Dew, 2000). Many of the residential centers that include animals in their programs have dogs.

Cats: Cats are good animals to include in the therapeutic process because they are independent to a point and can remain at the office at night and on weekends if the counselor so desires. The late Boris Levinson, Ph.D., used his own cat, Juanita, to illustrate examples with his patients.

Rabbits, Guinea Pigs, and Pocket Pets: Rabbits, guinea pigs, and pocket pets are animals that clients may hold and pet. The smaller pocket pets, including the reptiles, will most likely create attention amongst the smaller children and adolescent boys. Rabbits, guinea pigs, and the cuddly pocket pets work well when the client needs to hold or touch something. Many of the topics discussed in the previous section would work well incorporated with these smaller animals.

Horses: Hippotherapy and therapeutic horseback riding are interventions with recreational and social benefits for individuals with chronic illness and disabilities (All and Loving, 1999). All and Loving (1999) also say that hippotherapy, a term derived from the Latin word hippos, meaning horse, is horseback riding used as a form of treatment, with specific predetermined goals of therapy. Therapeutic riding simply uses the recreational pleasures of horseback riding to promote various social, emotional, and physical benefits (Britton, cited in All & Loving, 1999, pg. 6).

Water Animals: The water animals are becoming more popular in the field of AAT. Jabs (1994) says that the fish's smooth underwater undulations [wavelike motions] have a calming effect on grown-ups as well. Gazing into the aquarium somehow makes the wait for shots or test results a little easier to take. In a recent experiment, by Dr. Katcher, watching a video tape of tropical fish proved more absorbing and relaxing than watching a tank full of real fish, judging from measurements of blood pressure (Vines, 1994). This study suggests that the bright color of the fish attract the human eye more than the plain colored fish.

<u>Dolphins:</u> Dolphins have been used within the counseling process for several decades now. They have been very effective with developmentally disabled people, especially children. Cerullo (1999) says that researchers have found that children with disabilities who are allowed to interact with dolphins often make great strides in their therapy.

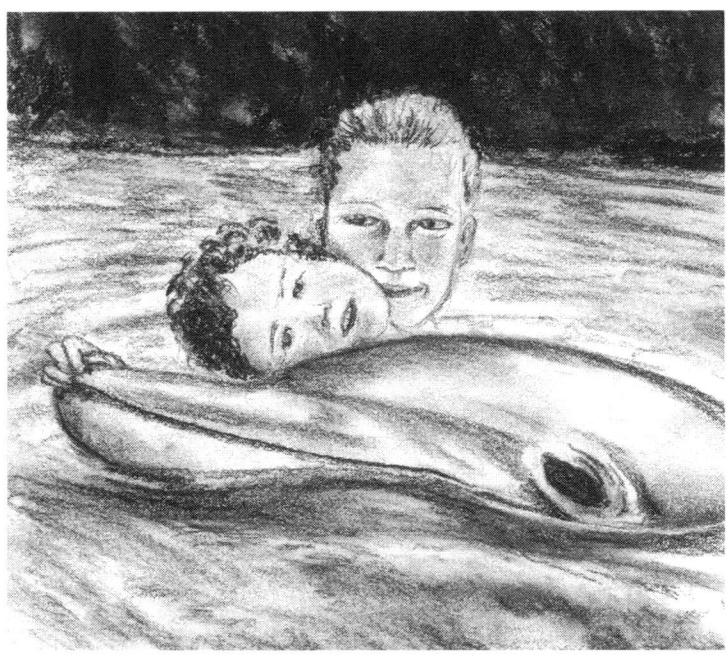

Maria Steurer is a dolphin trainer at Dolphin Reef in Eilat, Israel, in a part of the Red Sea. The dolphins are more gentle with disabled people, as if they sense that there is something special about them, says Steurer (Cerullo, 1999). She has seen many seriously ill people, especially children, make impressive gains after petting, swimming with, and befriending dolphins (Cerullo, 1999).

<u>Farm Animals:</u> In Lima, Ohio, at a facility for mentally ill inmates, part of the courtyard resembles a barnyard (Toufexis, 1987). Sheep, goats, ducks, rabbits, even deer, roam around. "We're finding the prisoners who have pets are less violent," says Psychiatric Social Worker David Lee (Toufexis, 1987).

Basic Tenets of AAT

Basic tenets are provided by Green Chimney's Children's Services and Susan Brooks, Psy. D. Dr. Brooks works in the farm and wildlife center. The following list was offered through their web-site at http://www.pcnet.com/~gchimney/interactions/interactions.htm.

1.   AAT is a triangular relationship; one that is dynamic and flowing.

2.   One must have respect of the animal as an animal. AAT does not anthropormorphize. You do not assign or project human emotions onto the animal. AAT does not "use" animals, but works in conjunction with the animal's basic temperament and capacities.

3.   AAT is cognizant of stress in the triangle, either from or towards the animal or humans.

4. The therapist involved in AAT must be knowledgeable of the history of each in the triangle…i.e. has the dog been fearful of slippery floors and become stressed walking down the hallway of a hospital?… or has the person you are working with have a history of abuse to animals in their past?

5. Therapists utilizing AAT must be aware and create a sense of balance in the dynamic and flowing triangular relationship.

6. Therapists utilizing AAT are aware of and concerned about safety issues at all times in the relationship with the person and for the animal.

7. The therapist establishes the boundaries which connect humans and animals as part of AAT. The therapist looks to the strengths and weaknesses of the animal as well as their personal issues as the coordinator of the triangle… i.e. if the therapist is asked to assist with grief counseling utilizing AAT and personally does not deal very well with death and dying, the therapist must realize that boundary in themselves. The therapist must know what one brings to the triangle at any given moment and how that energy impacts the dynamic flow of the triangle.

Ethical Issues

Some of the basic tenets from the Green Chimneys Children's Services, Inc. cross over into the realm of ethical issues. Ethical issues are very important because they provide the counselor with a basis for practicing correctly, and provide and preserve safety in the therapy sessions when used appropriately.

Fine (2000) says that the issue is how to balance the needs of human clients with respect for the needs of the animal. Aubrey H. Fine lists five basic ethical principles for use of the therapy animal in her book, Handbook on Animal-Assisted Therapy: Theoretical Foundations and Guidelines for Practice. These ethical principles include the following:

1. All animals utilized therapeutically must be kept free from abuse, discomfort, and distress, both physical and mental.

2. Proper health care for the animal must be provided at all times.

3. All animals should be capable of having a quiet place where they can have time away from their work activities. Clinicians must practice preventive health procedures for all animals.

4. Interactions with clients must be structured so as to maintain the animal's capacity

to serve as a useful therapeutic agent.

5.   A situation of abuse or stress for a therapy animal should never be allowed except in such cases where temporarily permitting such abuse is necessary to avoid a serious injury to or abuse of the human client.

Fine (2000) offers procedures for ethical decision making regarding therapy animals and implications of procedure for ethical decision making regarding therapy animals. This researcher strongly recommends that the reader who is seriously interested in AAT either acquire this book from a library or buy the book at a local bookstore or through the internet.

The therapist or facility that integrates animals into the counseling process must become educated about the animal(s) that he or she is working with. Animals have unique diets and needs that must be provided for. Some animals cannot remain by themselves over a weekend because they must be fed daily. If they aren't, they may starve or become malnourished. Fish must not be overcrowded and phosphorus and ammonia levels must be appropriate or they will die. Dolphins must have plenty of space, water, and appropriate diet to remain healthy and happy in captivity. Farm animals need to move around and graze, as well as horses. Smaller animals that live in cages need to exercise out of their cages on a regular basis. Certain animals need more affection from people than others do.

It is crucial that the therapist or facility prepare themselves ahead of time. They must do research and decide which animal(s) are best suited for their facility. All animals must be taken care of properly.

Examples of Animal Integration

Hamsters: Bob B. was nine years old. He viciously attacked children and teachers and had been expelled from several schools, felt worthless, brought food from school home because he thought that was the only food not poisoned, trusted no one, and was infantilized by his family because another child had died in his father's arms (Levinson, revised by Mallon, 1997, p. 114). He longed for a hamster, and at school was permitted to adopt one, which had great therapeutic value for him (Levinson, revised by Mallon, 1997, p. 114). Note Bob's progress after acquiring the hamster from the book Pet-Oriented Child Psychotherapy:

He learned that in order to survive without its mother, the hamster had to depend upon him and to trust him. This was something Bob had great difficulty with himself. He began to see that this was not altogether an impossible idea. For example, the hamster actually ate the food Bob gave him—and not just one kind of food, but any kind that Bob gave him. Bob could plainly see that the hamster was not poisoned, and it was food different from the cheese sandwich that he had been eating daily for months. Bob also saw that on rare occasions, when he was absent or unable to feed the hamster, others performed this task—and much to Bob's amazement the hamster did not die. Thus, he came to trust a tiny bit and to dispel slightly his food poisoning fantasy. In addition, Bob was very frightened at first that the hamster would fall off the tabletop where we were training the animal to become friendly with Bob. Bob was sure that if the hamster did fall, he would die. One day, the hamster did fall. And miracle of miracle, it did not die. Bob was surprised, pleased, and began to show some signs of relinquishing his catastrophic expectations of life. He began to take a few more chances himself. He even assured his parents that he was capable of taking care of the hamster, that nothing would happen to it if he cared for it; that his mother who considered it dirty and was afraid of it was not to take

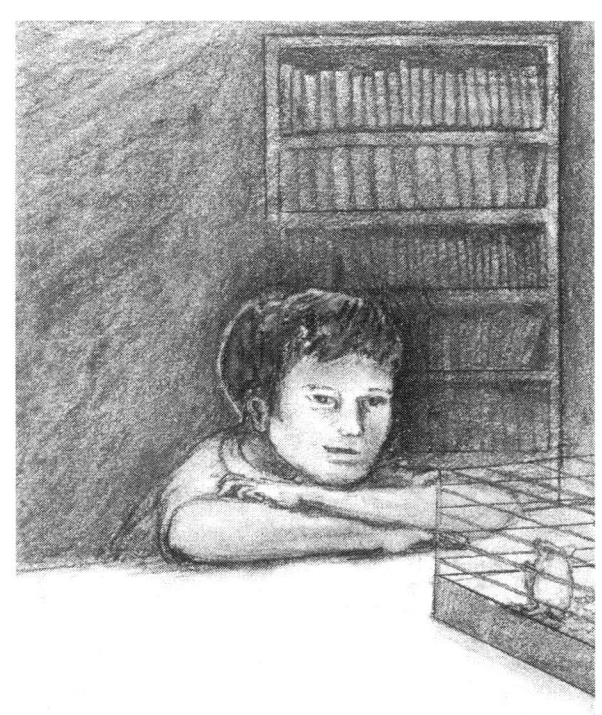

care of it; but that he would show her how to handle it. This turnabout of roles was good for Bob. For once, he was the capable one. Bob, who brooded over the belief that he was worthless because he had never done anything for anyone, began to feel a little more value as a person. He began to separate himself ever so slightly from parental hold. Bob's mother learned to like the hamster and at least, out of respect for Bob, to refrain from calling it dirty. The acquisition of the hamster also had a beneficial influence on his school behavior. Because Bob was a violent, hysterical child, with frequent outbursts of kicking, spitting, biting, swearing, and running out of the school, it was difficult to retain him in a classroom without an aide for five hours a day, five days a week with four other disturbed boys. His hamster provided real therapy for him when he had been untractable by any other method. (Levinson, revised by Mallon, 1997, p. 114-115)

Gerbils: In the book, Once Upon a Time…Therapeutic Stories That Teach & Heal, Nancy Davis uses symbols and metaphors through storytelling. Davis (1996) says that symptoms of PTSD keep a child "stuck" with a need to control. Davis (1996) also says that it is time to find a way out of your circular thinking, and leave the prison which your need to control has created.

Davis discusses the gerbil's cage door being locked from the inside. Davis (1996) says that the message is that the person in the cage has the power to find a way out. The gerbil running on the exercise wheel symbolizes the circular thinking and being "stuck" characteristic of PTSD (Davis, 1996). The gerbil finding a way to unlock the door symbolizes the challenge to the unconscious to find other ways to cope and to feel safe (Davis, 1996). The cage symbolizes the isolation of withdrawing from others which is also characteristic of PTSD (Davis, 1996).

These symbols and metaphors can help children and adults to work through various issues in the counseling process. Davis (1996) says after the therapist made up a Gerbil Story with the boy, the mother left it on the car seat. He found the following story on the seat of the car, riding home from therapy (Davis, 1996). Davis (1996) also says that she called very excited several days later to report that her son had been sleeping through the night and his mood was much improved. Animals can be used through symbols and metaphors in storytelling. The therapist may combine storytelling with the integration of an animal.

Water Animals: Boris Levinson had an aquarium in his waiting room. Some children watch the antics of the fish and weave many a fantasy which later may be played out in the therapy session (Levinson, revised by Mallon, 1997, p. 71). The aquarium may be a potent projective device, (…) personify some feared fantasy object, and (…) permits to child to bridge the land of his imagination [unconscious] with that of reality (Levinson, revised by Mallon, 1997, p. 71).

Levinson, revised by Mallon, 1997, p. 71, says that some children are afraid to grow, to develop, and to mature since growth symbolized leaving the dependent childish state and becoming responsible for one's self and one's actions. Observations of the fish in the aquarium and discussion of their growth and development may help a child to see his own misgivings in their true light (Levinson, revised by Mallon, 1997, p. 71).

Cats: With regard to using pets for illustrative purposes with patients in psychotherapy, my latest and third cat, Juanita, (…) was extremely frightened of human beings when she came to live with me (Levinson, revised by Mallon, 1997, p. 164). The explanation of Juanita's change from a frightened young cat who shrank away when you approached to pet her to a very receptive cat who actually approaches now for petting and "smooths" up against my patients is quite analogous to the way I teach my patients to change, and I use Juanita as an example of how they will change when I explain psychotherapy to them in the first therapy session (Levinson, revised by Mallon, 1997, p. 164).

Farm Animals: Primarily, the benefits derive from children learning how to handle animals, to develop a relationship with them and through them with nature which can expedite healing (Levinson, revised by Mallon, 1997, p. 98). Those who were previously unable to join in any communal effort may find themselves motivated by animals to participate in work committees assigned to the care of animals (Levinson, revised by Mallon, 1997, p. 99). The need to make choices and decision's for the institution's pets can strengthen weak egos and foster cooperation among the children (Levinson, revised by Mallon, 1997, p. 99).

Horses: As was stated earlier in the horse section of this research paper, therapeutic riding simply uses the recreational pleasures of horseback riding to promote various social, emotional, and physical benefits (All and Loving, 1999). Due to the wide range of issues and health concerns that a client may have, it may be necessary that the therapist refer the client to a hippotherapist. Hippotherapists are specially trained physical therapists, occupational therapists, or both, who utilize horseback riding as a therapeutic modality (Jorgenson, 1997; National Institute for Health, 1987, cited in All and Loving, 1999, p.6).

These studies focused on children and adults with a variety of disabilities, such as spinal cord impairment, CVA, head injury, cerebral palsy, blindness, deafness, multiple sclerosis, spina bifida, polio, autism, mental retardation, psychiatric problems, and learning disabilities (Brudvig, 1988; Freeman, 1984; Griffith, 1992; Potter et al., 1994, cited in All and Loving, 1999, p.7).

Dogs:

1. Companionship

A young woman responded that her sister and the company of her two dogs were the most helpful in dealing with her loss and difficulty with anxiety "[When I had] panic at night, my dogs [were the] only things that helped (Sable, 1995). I sat on the floor with them. [They're] just being there" (Sable, 1995). The presence of these dogs made a difference in coping with the loss of her husband and her husband's dog due to death.

2. Rapport

Toufexis (1987) says that troubled teenagers, for example, are more likely to open up when a therapist brings a dog along. In the article Furry and Feathery Therapists, Toufexis writes:

Carol Antoinette Peacock, a psychologist in Watertown, Mass., starts treatment of new adolescent patients with an introduction to her dog Toffy. "It helps them to trust me," says Peacock, who finds that patients sometimes express their feelings through the animal. They'll say, 'Your dog looks pretty sad,' meaning 'I'm pretty sad.' (Toufexis, 1987, p. 74)

3. <u>Disclosure:</u>

Reichert (1998) says that children often project their feelings about themselves onto the animal, which gives love, does not talk back or argue, and provides a continuous nonjudgmental relationship. A child often finds it easier to express herself through physical interaction with the animal, rather than verbal communication (Reichert, 1998). The social worker encourages the child to tell her sexual abuse story to the animal being used in the session (Reichert, 1998). The child began telling Buster about how the child's uncle had hurt her private parts (Reichert, 1998). Throughout the story, the child held Buster's paw and continued to hold and pet Buster after she had finished telling her story (Reichert, 1998). In the article <u>Individual Counseling for Sexually Abused Children: A Role for Animals and Storytelling</u>, Reichert writes:

When using stories, the social worker needs to tailor the story to the child's issues. The child was a seven-year old boy whose older brother, age 10, had already disclosed that a neighbor had sexually abused both of them. To help the child express his feelings and tell what had happened to him, the author told the following story (adopted from Davis, 1990):

Once upon a time, there was a doggie named Buster. Buster lived with her mommy and two brothers and was very happy. She loved to play, especially when she got to run in the woods, meet other doggies and chase squirrels. One day, Buster disappeared in the woods for awhile and when she returned, she was different. She was afraid of everything, wet her bed, and had tummy aches. Her family saw that she was scared. They asked her, "What is wrong, Buster?" But Buster couldn't say anything because she had gotten an invisible, magic bandage over her mouth while she was in the woods. Buster was afraid that if she took it off, something bad would happen. A few days later, Buster got a splinter in her tail. Buster could not tell her mommy about the splinter because the invisible bandage was still over Buster's mouth. Then an old dog tried to bully Buster. The old dog said, "I bet you can't even swim." Buster thought to herself, "That dog is wrong." Buster went to a pond and swam across it. The old dog had tried to trick Buster, who was a very smart dog. Now Buster started to think about the invisible, magic bandage. "I bet it's a trick, too!," she said to herself as she pulled it off. Nothing bad happened. Buster ran home and told her mommy all about the woods and what had happened there. The more Buster told her mommy about the woods, the safer and more powerful she felt. Buster also told her mommy about the splinter. Buster's mommy helped Buster get the splinter out of Buster's tail. From then on, Buster was

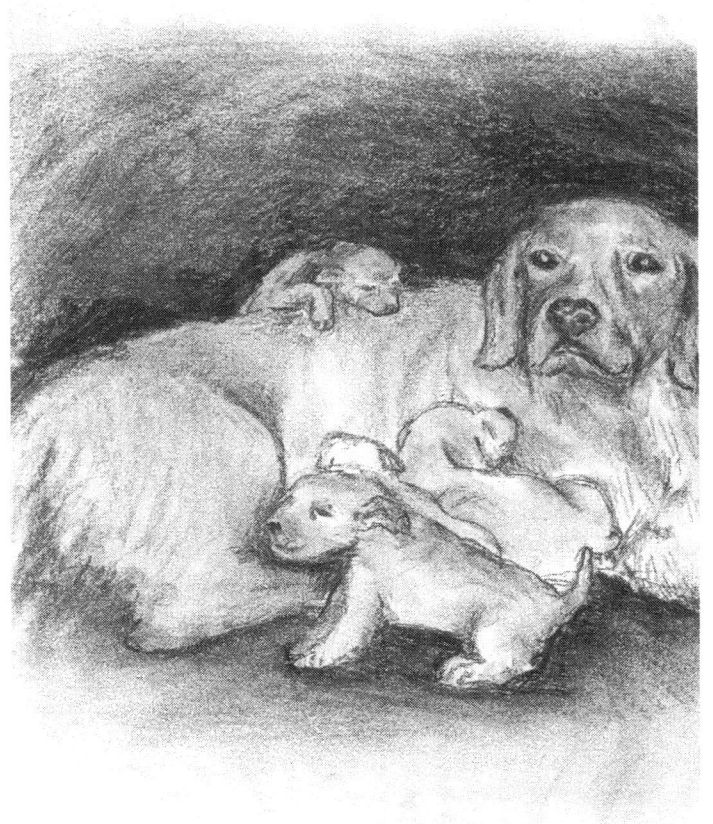

not afraid to sleep, and Buster's tummy felt better. Buster had figured out that the invisible magic bandage wasn't magic at all. The bandage was there to simply keep her quiet. Buster had learned a lesson she would always remember. Telling the truth about trips in the woods to grown ups who help children made her feel strong and safe. (Reichert, 1998, p. 183)

Reichert (1998) says that after telling the story, the author asked the child the following questions: How do you think Buster felt coming out of the woods with an invisible, magic bandage on her mouth? How do you think Buster felt after taking off the bandage? How do you think Buster feels now? In the next session, the child disclosed the sexual abuse by his neighbor (Reichert, 1998). During this disclosure, the child held Buster (Reichert, 1998).

    4. <u>Shame and guilt:</u>

Children often experience shame and guilt about sexual abuse (Gil, Marvasati, & James, cited in Reichert, 1998, pg. 184). Sometimes children believe that they brought on the abuse because they feel they did something wrong and the abuse was their fault (Reichert, 1998). To help children express feelings regarding shame and guilt, the author told the following story, also involving Buster (Reichert, 1998). Reichert also writes:

> Once upon a time I heard a mournful cry outside my house. I thought it was the neighbor's dog first, but the crying kept on and on. So I went outside and there was a puppy named Buster, who was scared and frightened and all covered with fleas and ticks. Someone had put Buster there and left her all by herself. Buster thought she had been put on the wrong side of the road because she had cheated in school and she knew that was wrong. (Reichert, 1998, p. 184)

The social worker usually ends the story with the phrase "bad things can happen to good little doggies like Buster just as bad things can happen to good little kids" (Reichert, 1998). Reichert (1998) says that the social worker can then ask the child the following question: Whose fault was it that Buster was put on the side of the road? The child can then respond to the story, and the social worker and child can address issues of guilt and responsibility (Reichert, 1998).

Storytelling in animal assisted therapy helps the child disclose the abuse and express feelings (Reichert, 1998). By integrating the animal into the story, the social worker presents the child with the opportunity to identify with the animal and project her feelings onto the animal, thus facilitating disclosure and expression of feelings (Reichert, 1998).

5. Expression of feeling:

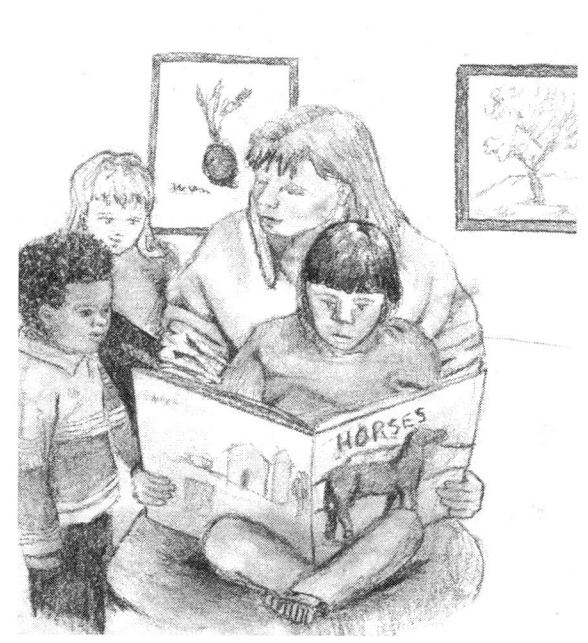

In, "Throwaway" Kids and "Throwaway" Animals Found Each Other, Lansdell discusses how the teenagers in the group home began to feel (cited in Anderson and Anderson, 1999). Lansdell says that the director showed the students graphic pictures of animal abuse and neglect that touched even the young males, who had done time in prison and were proud of it (cited in Anderson and Anderson, 1999). It wasn't unusual to see them quickly brush away tears (Lansdell, cited in Anderson and Anderson, 1999, p. 88). Later, they'd write in their daily journals for me to read about feelings that were too private and tender for them to express openly (Lansdell, cited in Anderson and Anderson, 1999, p. 88).

The director's visits and their growing concern for the animals opened a small window for my kids to face the pain and shame they'd endured as survivors of abuse (Lansdell, cited in Anderson and Anderson, 1999, p. 88). Some students even did artwork for the shelter and wrote poems trying to express the animals' inner feelings and yearning for loving families. Lansdell says that all the animals served to touch these young hearts, opening them to give and receive love (cited in Anderson and Anderson, 1999).

Becoming Certified

Delta Society offers classes to the professional who wants to become certified as an AAT specialist. Delta Society's headquarters are located in Renton, Washington. Delta Society (2001) says that people who wish to work as an Animal-Assisted Therapy Specialist must first be credentialed in their field of choice (nursing, social work, counseling, teaching, physical therapy, occupational therapy, recreational therapy, etc.). Many of the positions utilizing these degrees require a masters degree in order to practice therapy (Delta Society, 2001).

The professional may receive a degree or certificate in AAT from other places as well, including colleges, universities, centers, and associations throughout the country. Delta Society provides a resource list of them. However, Delta Society is the leading provider of credentials and continuing education related to AAT (Delta Society, 2001).

To be considered AAT, a professional must use the animal as part of his or her own specialty (Delta Society, 2001). For example, a social worker must use the animal in the context of social work (Delta Society, 2001). The animal is integrated directly into the client's treatment plan. The professional identifies and defines the goals before the session begins, and documents the session's progress and activity (Delta Society, 2001). This is how animal-assisted therapy may facilitate the counseling process and create a positive affect upon the therapy.

Summary

Children, adolescents, adults, and elderly may benefit from the integration of animals into the client's therapeutic program. Integration of the animal will benefit both the client and professional. Many benefits may result, which creates a win-win situation for both the client and therapist.

There are various facilities where AAT can be used. Different animals will work best in different facilities. It is crucial that the therapist and/or facility learns how to take proper care of the animal(s). Applications and uses of AAT are plentiful, as well as the animals that may be used in the therapeutic setting. Many different animals may be integrated into the client's treatment plan that may include various psychological and behavioral issues.

The basic tenets and ethical issues must be considered and followed through. These are necessary so that the triangle may function properly and be safe for each member. The triangle includes the therapist, client, and animal. Becoming certified may be accomplished through various programs, schools, and organizations throughout the country. This concludes the literature-based guidebook.

CHAPTER 3

METHODOLOGY

Introduction

The purpose of this study was to develop a literature based guide on the use of animal-assisted therapy for the clinical, school, and educational counselors who wish to incorporate animal-assisted therapy into their work with clients. Social workers who work within the realm of counseling and referral networking may benefit also. The research question was stated as 'What is the content of a literature-based guidebook on the use of animal-assisted therapy?'

Research Design

The design of this study was descriptive in nature. The study's purpose was to describe and integrate the facts and characteristics of current and past literature, the population and animals involved, and related areas of interest. Literature was investigated and incorporated into the formation of a consolidated guidebook. Descriptive design suited this research project the best because the data in the literature incorporated had to be explained, integrated, and organized into this guidebook.

Method of Analysis

This researcher collected data from professional journals, books, health and psychological magazines, and organizations. The data was analyzed so that appropriate literature was included into this research project. This researcher organized the data so that the reader may learn, understand, and have access to further avenues if additional interest in animal-assisted therapy results.

Assumptions and Limitations

Some assumptions should be noted and explained. The term "use" of the animal in this guidebook was not intended in a derogatory or negative way. The term "use" had more to do with integration and explanation of how to include the animal in the therapeutic process.

This guidebook contained a contrast of the term projection by two different authors in the research. It should be understood that there is good and bad projection onto the animal. It is good to project the client's feelings by saying, "the dog is sad" when the client is really sad. It is bad projection when any form of abuse occurs and the client or therapist literally tries to make the animal feel the client's feelings and go through what the client went through. This would be unethical.

Some limitations have resulted. All of the animals cannot be included within the scope of this research project. The reader should not assume that the animals listed are the only animals that can be integrated into the client's counseling process. With appropriate training and creativity, additional animals may be integrated.

Some clients will have allergic reactions to certain types of animals. These clients must be around hairless animals, water animals, or reptiles. The client's health must be preserved.

Other clients will have a fear or dislike of animals. Animal-assisted therapy would not be appropriate with those client populations, unless the client specifically wanted to work on his or her fear of animals. Then that could be incorporated into a treatment plan with some form of desensitization.

This researcher is fond of all animals, however that did not cause bias within this research study. Literature was collected from various sources, analyzed, and integrated where appropriate. The data results were cited properly. The literature was unanimously positive concerning integrating animals into the counseling process.

CHAPTER 4

SUMMARY, CONCLUSIONS, AND RECOMMENDATIONS

Summary

The focus of this study was to develop a guidebook that will educate mental health professionals about the use of AAT. This guidebook included populations that can benefit from AAT, benefits to the client and clinician, facilities where AAT may be used, specific applications and uses of AAT, animal species used in AAT, basic tenets and ethical issues, examples of animal integration, and certification.

The purpose of this study was to develop a literature based guidebook on the use of AAT for the clinical, school, and educational counselors who wish to incorporate animal-assisted therapy into their work with clients. Social workers who work within the realm of counseling and referral networking may benefit also.

The literature review consolidated literature that has been done by therapists, organizations, training centers, authors, and editors. The literature discussed a variety of animals and gave examples on how to integrate the animal. The findings showed that AAT is beneficial to the client and therapist, promotes healing and progress in the therapeutic sessions, and is a positive experience as long as the guidelines, ethical issues, and proper animal is integrated into the process. Respect must be given to the animal as well.

Conclusions and Recommendations

It should be noted that clinicians in all fields, including nurses and occupational, physical, and recreational therapists may practice as an animal-assisted therapist. Psychiatric nurses often provide counseling as well as other nursing duties.

The therapist who wishes to integrate animals into the client's treatment plan must understand the following. An animal-assisted therapist must be comfortable with the animal that he or she selects. The therapist must do research and find out how to take proper care of that animal and understand that he or she will take responsibility for the animal's needs, such as exercise, health care, play time, need for attention, etc. Unless the residential center agrees to take on the responsibility of the animal, the therapist will be the animal's owner.

Animals may benefit from the therapeutic process. The animal has an opportunity to have a good home, get attention and love, and be taken care of properly. Animals may be adopted from the local animal shelters and used in therapy rather than be put to sleep because there aren't enough homes available for them. Purebred animals may also be utilized.

The therapist cannot use any animal. The animal must get along well with strangers petting and holding him or her. The animal's personality must work well in the therapeutic setting. The animal must fit the criteria of an animal-assisted training facility's expectations. A therapist who takes in his or her own pet once in a while is not an animal-assisted therapist unless he or she becomes certified in AAT.

Implementing and designing an AAT program, liability, cost-effectiveness, and infection control issues are topics that must be researched after the therapist becomes seriously interested in becoming an animal-assisted therapist. These topics and many others can be researched in greater detail in the book, <u>Handbook on Animal-Assisted</u>

<u>Therapy: Theoretical Foundations And Guidelines For Practice</u>, edited by Aubrey H. Fine.

Referrals must be given when the therapist cannot handle a topic, has unresolved personal issues concerning the topic, or does not have the education or training concerning that topic. Remember, the animal is only integrated as one tool in the treatment planning process. The animal is not magic and cannot provide the only means of healing. Work must still be done by the client and therapist.

To remain current in the field of AAT, this researcher suggests that the therapist become a member of an organization such as the Delta Society. This will allow the researcher to network with other mental health workers, such as therapists, school counselors, and social workers. Organizations provide valuable information on their specific field of expertise. The therapist may continue to learn about resources such as books, journals, and other facilities and organizations.

Appendix A will follow the listing of references. The appendix will provide the therapist with resources that he or she may use to take the next steps in the process of becoming an animal-assisted therapist.

REFERENCE LIST

All, A. and Loving, G. (1999). Animals, horseback riding, and implications for rehabilitation therapy. <u>Journal of Rehabilitation, 65</u>(3), 49-57.

Altschuler, E.L. (1999). Pet-facilitated therapy for posttraumatic stress disorder. <u>Annals of Clinical Psychiatry, 11</u>(1) 29-30.

Anderson, A. and Anderson, L. (1999). Angel Animals. New York: Penguin Putnam Inc.

Bardill, N. and Hutchinson, S. (1997). Animal-assisted therapy with hospitalized adolescents. <u>Journal of Child and Adolescent Psychiatric Nursing, 10</u>(1) 17-24.

Black, S. (1996). Helping depressed students. <u>Education Digest, 62</u>(1) 53-56.

Bruck, L. (1996). Today's ancillaries, Part 2: Art, music, and pet therapy. <u>Nursing Homes Long Term Care Management, 45</u>(7) 36-43.

Burke, S. (1992). In the presence of animals. <u>U.S. News & World Report, 112</u>(7) 64-65.

Cerullo, M. (1999). Dolphins: What They Can Teach Us. New York: Dutton Children's Books.

Connor, K. and Miller, J. (2000). Help from our animal friends. <u>Nursing Management, 31</u> (7) 42, 44-46.

Davis, N. (1996). Once upon a time…therapeutic stories that teach & heal. Maryland:

Nancy Davis.

Delta Society. (2001). (petsforum.com/deltasociety/dsj100.htm).

Delta Society. (1997). <u>Animal-assisted therapy. Therapeutic interventions</u>. Washington: Author.

Dew, B. (2000). Co-therapy with Moses. <u>Family Journal, 8</u>(2) 199-202.

Dog World. (2000). <u>Study on pet bond and therapy funded</u>. Colorado: Author.

Dzikowski, D. (1998). Saltwater aquariums provide deep-sea-style stress relief. <u>Westchester County Business Journal, 37</u>(23) 24-5.

Fine, A. (2000). Handbook on animal-assisted therapy. Theoretical foundations and guidelines for practice. New York: Academic Press.

Gammonley, J., Howie, A., Kirwin, S., Zapf, S., Frye, J., Freeman, G., Stuart-Russell, R. (1997). Animal-assisted therapy: therapeutic interventions. Washington: Delta Society.

Golin, M. and Walsh, T. (1994). Heal emotions with fur, feathers and love. <u>Prevention, December</u> 81-3.

Green Chimneys Children's Services, Inc. (2001). (www.pcnet.com/~gchimney/interactions/interactions.htm).

Jabs, C. (1994). Fish without strings. <u>Country Living, 17</u>(8) 130-1.

Janssen, M. (1998). Therapeutic interventions: animal assisted therapy programs. <u>Palaestra, 14</u>(4) 40.

Kindsvater, L. (1999). Canines provide therapy for hospice patients. <u>Las Vegas Business Press, 16</u>(18) 15.

Kowalski, G. (1991,1999). The Souls of Animals. Novato, CA: New World Library.

Levinson, B. and Mallon, G. (1997). Pet-oriented child psychotherapy. Springfield, IL: Charles C. Thomas Publishers, Ltd.

Netting, F., Wilson, C., & New, J. (1987). The human-animal bond: implications for practice. <u>Social Work, 32</u>(1) 60-4.

Reichert, E. (1998). Individual counseling for sexually abused children: a role for animals and storytelling. <u>Child and Adolescent Social Work Journal, 15</u>(3) 177-85.

Sable, Pat. (1995). Pets, attachment, and well-being across the life cycle. <u>Social Work,</u> <u>40</u>(3) 334-41.

Siegel, M. (1995). The power of pets. <u>Good Housekeeping, 221</u>(5) 26.

Toufexis, A. (1987). Furry and feathery therapists. <u>Time, 129</u>(13) 74.

Trivedi, L., and Perl, J. (1995). Animal facilitated counseling in the elementary school: a literature review and practical considerations. <u>Elementary School Guidance &</u> <u>Counseling, 29</u>(3) 223-34.

Vines, G. (1994). The astounding healing power of pets. <u>Health Confidential, 8</u>(6) 9-11.

Whispering Hope Ranch. Brochure. (www.whisperinghoperanch.org)

Whitaker, J. (1994). Adopt a pet for your own good health. <u>Human Events, 50</u>(27) 8.

APPENDIX A

LIST OF AAT RESOURCES

APPENDIX A:

LIST OF AAT RESOURCES

Organizations

Animals Benefit Club of Arizona Inc.
3111 East Saint John Road
Phoenix, AZ 85032
(602) 867/2169
www.animalsbenefitclub.com
No kill animal shelter, trains and certifies animal assisted therapy teams.

Delta Society
289 Perimeter Road East
Renton, WA 98055-1329
(425) 226-7357
http://www.deltasociety.org
Provides information, training, certification, information on training programs throughout the country, articles, and books

Therapy Dogs International, Inc.
88 Bartley Road
Flanders, NJ 07836
(973) 252-9800 office
(973) 252-7171 fax
www.tdi-dog.org
Provides qualified handlers and their therapy dogs for visits, training, and testing programs.

Facilities

Green Chimneys Children's Services, Inc.
Residential treatment center
Brewster, New York
info@greenchimneys.com

Whispering Hope Ranch
HC2 Box 162-V
Payson, AZ 85541
(520) 478-0410 fax/phone
www.whisperinghoperanch.org

The Human Dolphin Institute
118 Treasure Palms Dr.
Panama City Beach, FL 32408
(850) 872-8003
(850) 234-7019
(850) 234-6748 fax
Email: info@human-dolphin.org

Dolphin Research Center
58901 Overseas Highway
Grassy Key, FL 33050-6019 USA
(305) 289-1121 office
(305) 743-7627 fax

Books

Animal-Assisted Therapy: Therapeutic Interventions
Delta Society, 1997
Contains many valuable resources

Handbook on Animal-Assisted Therapy:
Theoretical Foundations And Guidelines For Practice
Edited by Aubrey H. Fine
Academic Press, New York, 2000

Pets & Mental Health
Odean Cusack, 1988
Discusses pets, mental health problems, and how the two relate

Internet Sites

http://www.dolphins.org/learn/dh_thrpy.htm

Journals and Periodicals

Anthrozoos, A Multidisciplinary Journal of the Interactions of People and Animals.
Quarterly. Purdue University Press.
1207 SCC-E West Lafayette, Indiana, 47907-1207
1-800-933-9637
libpup@omni.cc.purdue.edu

ADDITIONS SINCE ANIMAL ASSISTED THERAPY WAS WRITTEN

Facilities

Whispering Hope Ranch, in Payson, Arizona, hosts camps and retreats for children and adults. The ranch now hosts retreats for adults as well as children with mental and physical illnesses and disabilities. The ranch has lodging and dining and provides access to individuals with disabilities. Individual tours have now ceased and the focus in on camps and retreats.

The new numbers to Whispering Hope Ranch are: 928-478-0339 phone 928-478-0410 fax

The Joyful Heart Foundation is a foundation started by the actress Mariska Hargitay in 2002. Talk, art, and dolphin/human therapy are provided to victims of rape and sexual abuse.

There website is: www.joyfulheartfoundation.org.

Organizations

The new address of the Delta Society is:

875 124th Ave NE, Ste 101 Bellevue, WA 98005-2531 425-679-5500 phone 425-679-5539 fax
info@deltasociety.org

Internet Sites

Dolphin assisted therapy information can be found at: www.specialchild.com.

Green Chimneys can be located at: www.greenchimneys.org.

The Dolphin Research Center can be located at:
drc@dolphins.org
www.dolphins.org

Additional Information

Charles C. Thomas, Publisher, Ltd., transferred copyright back to Boris Levinson, the author of Pet-oriented child psychotherapy. Since then, Boris Levinson has passed away.

The Human Dolphin Institute in Panama City Beach, Florida, cannot be found through mail or internet.

The author Lynda M. King would like to advise individuals of the following. Before obtaining a pet for pleasure or for utilization in therapy, do research and learn how to properly care for the animal or mammal. Make sure the pet will be a good match for the individual or individuals who will be caring for the pet. The children and adult sections of a local library, a pet store, a breeder or trainer, and the internet are excellent sources to learn how to properly care for an animal or mammal.

About the Book

This book will provide the reader with a well rounded understanding of animal-assisted therapy, or "pet therapy." Animal-assisted therapy is a therapeutic tool that is used to facilitate the client's treatment and recovery process. Some of the people who will benefit from reading this book include counselors, school counselors, social workers, educators, students, and anyone interested in animal-assisted therapy. Teachers may implement this book in their instructional materials.

Authors, books, journals, articles, and resources have been consolidated into a descriptive designed graduate level thesis. There is a detailed table of contents that will allow the reader to quickly access the section he or she is looking for. A glossary consisting of animal-assisted therapy topics is provided. This book reads easily and will engage the reader.

Ways to integrate land and marine mammals into the client's treatment will be shown, as well as the kinds of land and marine mammals to be utilized. Animal-assisted therapy may be utilized with many clinical diagnoses and therapeutic issues. There are many types of facilities that may benefit from animal-assisted therapy. Examples and further explanation will be given addressing these topics.

Basic tenets, ethical issues, and certification will be explained. Within the helping professions, ethics are vital and certification has become mandatory in many states. The needs of the client, the clinician, and the animal will be discussed. Benefits of animal-assisted therapy will be included.

Resources that will facilitate the implementation of animal-assisted therapy will be shown. The reader who would like to pursue animal-assisted therapy in further detail will be given additional resources. The goal of this descriptive designed graduate level thesis was to consolidate many good works into one book. As time advances, the material presented in this book will continue to be useful.

BIOGRAPHICAL SKETCH

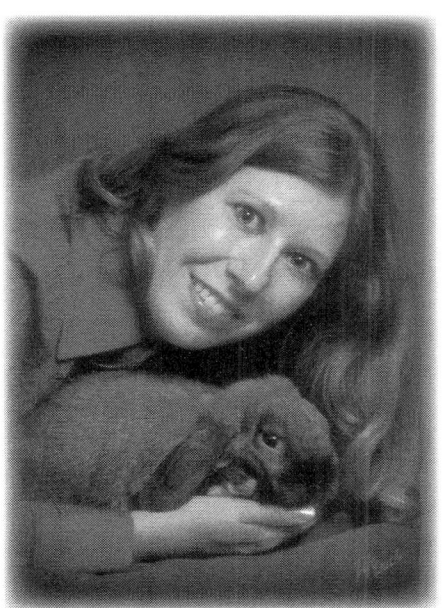

Lynda M. King, MAPC LAC, has facilitated animal-assisted therapy with Cody, her Holland Lop rabbit. They are also a registered pet partner's team.

Lynda M. King went to Tabor College in Hillsboro, Kansas. She completed an experimental psychology project on the interaction between humans and the guinea pig, implementing her guinea pig, Browny. She completed internships at an elementary school, nursing home, and mental health center. She graduated with a Bachelor of Arts in Psychology.

Ms. King attended graduate school at Ottawa University, in Phoenix, Arizona.

She completed a Master's research project. The thesis compiled several good authors and animal-assisted therapy topics into one book. Ms. King interned at a domestic violence shelter and at an adolescent residential treatment center. She graduated from Ottawa University with a Master of Arts in Professional Counseling, and obtained licensure in the state of Arizona in 2004.

Ms. King worked as a therapist at a mental health center in Arizona. She worked with children, teenagers, and adults. She incorporated her Holland Lop rabbit, Cody, into several counseling sessions. A child who was working on issues of defiance and hygiene related well to Cody. Cody purposely tipped over his water bowl. The child appeared amazed when Ms. King corrected Cody appropriately. Cody would display acts of good hygiene, and the child would observe him. Cody also served as a positive reward system when the child had appropriate behavior. Ms. King was able to correlate Cody's behavior with the children's behavior and incorporate animal-assisted therapy into their treatment goals.

In 2006, Ms. King and Cody obtained certification through the Animals Benefit Club of Arizona/Pet Partners Delta Society and are now a registered pet partner's team.

Ms. King has affection for land and marine mammals. Ms. King especially enjoys dolphins, and participated in the "Trainer for a Day" program at SeaWorld in San Diego, California. She is interested in dolphin therapy. Lynda King can be contacted at talk21ynda@msn.com or at animal_assisted_therapy@yahoo.com.

Printed in Great Britain
by Amazon

57276338R10040